Index

**CHAPTER 1: EFFECTIVENESS OF HAND SANITIZERS FOR DISINFECTION ESPECIALLY DURING PERIODS OF CRISIS:** ..........................................................................................6

Difference between handwashing and hand sanitization: ...............7

Availability of commercial hand sanitizers: .....................................9

Importance of homemade hand sanitizers during the crisis: ........11

**CHAPTER 2: DIFFERENT TYPES OF HAND SANITIZERS 13**

Classification on the basis of alcohol: ............................................13

Classification on the basis of consistency: ....................................15

Classification on the basis of production: .....................................16

**CHAPTER 3: HOW TO MAKE HIGH-QUALITY HAND SANITIZER AT HOME WITH MINIMAL BURDEN:** ............19

STEP 1: GATHERING THE REQUIRED ITEMS .....................22

STEP 2: USING ALL THE NECESSARY PRECAUTIONS .....30

STEP 3: MEASURING THE CALCULATED AMOUNT OF NECESSARY ITEMS: ................................................................33

STEP 4: MIXING THE CALCULATED AMOUNT OF NECESSARY ITEMS ................................................................35

STEP 5: HOW TO STORE IN SAFE AND USEABLE CONTAINER .................................................................................37

**CHAPTER 4: SPECIFIC RECIPE OF MAKING HAND SANITIZER FOR LARGER POPULATION:** ............................... **38**

**CHAPTER 5: SPECIAL CONSIDERATIONS ON USING HOMEMADE HAND SANITIZER:** ............................................. **40**

Proper use of high-quality homemade hand sanitizer: ............. 41

**CHAPTER 6: PROPER HANDWASHING TECHNIQUE:** ....... **43**

Summary: ................................................................................ 44

# Homemade hand sanitizer

*A Simple Step-By-Step Guide on How to Make Your Antibacterial Hand Sanitizer to Protect Yourself from Infections caused by Viruses and Germs and Stay Healthy*

- EFFECTIVENESS OF HAND SANITIZERS FOR DISINFECTION ESPECIALLY DURING PERIODS OF CRISIS
- DIFFERENT TYPES OF HAND SANITIZERS
- HOW TO MAKE HAND SANITIZER AT HOME WITH MINIMAL BURDEN
- STEP 1: GATHERING THE REQUIRED ITEMS
- STEP 2: USING ALL THE NECESSARY PRECAUTIONS
- STEP 3: MEASURING THE CALCULATED AMOUNT OF NECESSARY ITEMS
- STEP 4: MIXING THE CALCULATED AMOUNT OF NECESSARY ITEMS
- STEP 5: HOW TO STORE IN SAFE AND USEABLE CONTAINER
- SPECIAL CONSIDERATIONS ON USING HOMEMADE HAND SANITIZER

# CHAPTER 1: EFFECTIVENESS OF HAND SANITIZERS FOR DISINFECTION ESPECIALLY DURING PERIODS OF CRISIS:

It is an important debate that some body parts are more prone to bacterial and viral infections, while some of them also a role as a reservoir of bacterial and viral growth and transfer. Hands in the human body play the most crucial roles in sensing, touching and reaching activities. The touch and sensitivity receptors are maximally present in our hands, and thus, it is the most sensitive area of our body when it comes to proprioception. It has the highest ability to sense the objects with the help of touching stimuli which are transferred to the brain and then interpreted. Unfortunately, bacteria and viruses are also present in the highest ratio on our hands as compared to other visible body parts. It is important to note that besides the presence of the highest numbers of sensitivity receptors, our hands don't have the ability to sense the presence of these bacteria and viruses. These are microorganisms which cannot be seen through the naked eye, and sensory receptors of the human body are unable to feel the presence of these virulent organisms. It is the biggest reason that these microorganisms remain unchecked while transferring from one person to another. The human body can only perceive them through signs and symptoms induced by the diseases which are caused by these microorganisms. A smart choice is to eliminate these bacteria and viruses from our hands and skin at the earliest, and thus it will help in the prevention of many deadly infectious diseases caused by these germs and viruses.

Hand sanitization means clearing hands from germs which can be bacteria, viruses, spores or fungi, which can cause infections by penetrating through the human body and start chains of reactions which lead to full-fledged diseases. These diseases can be transmittable, which means, other humans can also be infected by these bacteria and viruses from a primary infected person. Hand sanitization helps in eradication and killing of these fungi and germs and thus prevents the infections and transmissions at the earliest step of the infectious chain. Hand sanitization requires agents which can kill the germs effectively and it also incorporates some specific hand washing or rubbing techniques which are essential for the proper working of sanitization agents. It is essential that to cover these effects; hand sanitizers are classified on the basis of types, formation, production and usage. The classification system of hand sanitizers will be discussed in relevant chapters.

**Difference between handwashing and hand sanitization:**

Hand washing and hand sanitization are always misinterpreted as the same in respect of terminology and meaning. However, technically speaking, hand washing and hand sanitization are very different from one another. Following are the basic differences in both types:

*Hand washing*
1. Hand washing means the use of water with or without a disinfectant solution to achieve cleanliness of hands.

2. Hand washing is used when hands are dirty and contaminated with visible contamination. It is a method of choice in this case
3. Washing hands with water and an antiseptic solution are the most superior type of disinfection for hands.
4. It is the oldest technique to promote health and cleanliness while preventing many deadly infections and diseases.
5. The biggest limitation of hand washing is the difficulty when water is unavailable. So, other sources of disinfection should be carried out to achieve cleanliness in that case.

## *Hand sanitization:*

1. Hand sanitization doesn't involve water to promote the health cleanliness specifically for hands.
2. When hands are dirty and visibly contaminated, hand sanitizers cannot be used as the method of choice. Hand sanitizers are unable to remove the visible contamination on hands.
3. Hand sanitization is inferior to handwashing with water and antiseptic solution.
4. It is the most advance technique which uses many easy to use and comfortable to carry sanitization solutions to achieve the cleanliness of hands.
5. The biggest limitation of hand sanitization is the inability of hand sanitizers to remove the visible dirt and contamination

from hands. Moreover, hand sanitization is inferior to handwashing with water and antiseptic solution.

So, from the above debate, it is clearly understood that when possible, always choose hand washing over hand sanitization because it is a most superior type of technique to promote hand cleanliness and thus prevention of many deadly infections and diseases which are caused by highly virulent viruses and bacteria.

The technique of hand washing and hand sanitization are similar and will be covered in relevant chapters.

**Availability of commercial hand sanitizers:**

Hand sanitizers are superior to hand washing technique with respect to the affordability and ease of use because they need no water to get the job done. Hand sanitizers are sold in many easy to carry boxes and containers which can be carried even in pockets, and this makes its use very easy. Two or three drops of an alcohol-based liquid or foam hand sanitizer and proper rubbing on hands for 20 seconds is all it takes to kill nearly 99% of bacteria and viruses on hands. Commercially made hand sanitizers are widely distributed all over the world under thousands of brand names. The price range of a pocket hand sanitizer is very affordable.

However, this is not very true when it comes to a crisis situation, especially during curfews and lockdowns in which the production capacities of commercial industries decline to an alarming situation. During crises related to pandemics or epidemics in which nearly every country of the world highly suffers from deadly infections, the availability of hand sanitizers can decline to an alarming level. This increases the pressure on commercial production of these hand sanitizers because of increased consumption during infections. The panic buying and very disturbed production to consumption ratio can lead to unavailability of these hand sanitizers in the market.

The unavailability of hand sanitizers during infectious pandemics can be more dangerous to pandemic itself. The biggest strategy used by health authorities during pandemics and epidemics is to prevent the incurable and poorly controlled infections rather than treating them. The first line of action for a preventive strategy related to infections is to kill the bacteria and viruses before they enter the human immune system. The primary method to break this chain is to cover the face from a high quality homemade or commercially available face mask and by using proper handwashing/sanitization techniques. If the production of hand sanitizers declines and consumption increases, in any case, the hand sanitizers can be entirely eliminated from the markets and thus, the chances of disease spread can be increased to many hundred folds. This is an alarming situation, and immediate actions will be needed to control the infectious spread. Here lies the importance of homemade hand sanitizers which can be a perfect substitute during the periods of crisis and readily available. The techniques of formation of homemade hand sanitizers are elementary, and it can be made from the items of daily household use. This raises the importance of awareness about homemade hand sanitizers to much extent. In this book, all the tricks and techniques used in the formation of a homemade hand sanitizer will be discussed in details.

**Importance of homemade hand sanitizers during the crisis:**

The use of hand sanitizer for killing many deadly bacteria and viruses is established. Healthcare authorities recommend the use of hand sanitizers, especially in periods of crisis to prevent the spread of disease because prevention is better than cure. If the production of hand sanitizers declines and consumption increases, in any case, the hand sanitizers can be entirely eliminated from the markets and thus, the chances of disease spread can be increased to many hundred folds. This is an alarming situation, and immediate actions will be needed to control the infectious spread. Here lies the importance of homemade hand sanitizers which can be a perfect substitute during the periods of crisis and readily available. The techniques of formation of homemade hand sanitizers are straightforward, and it can be made from the items of daily household use. This raises the importance of awareness about homemade hand sanitizers to much extent.

Homemade hand sanitizers are easy to make and more readily available than the commercially made hand sanitizers. The effectiveness and mode of action of homemade hand sanitizers are hundred per cent the same as compared to commercially made hand sanitizers. It is important to check the quality, techniques and item used in homemade hand sanitizer to achieve the maximum antibacterial and antiviral activity. Homemade hand sanitizer when perfectly made and used can kill nearly 99% of bacteria and viruses in a single go when it is used for more than 20 seconds on hands.

Homemade hand sanitizer is no doubt an essential disinfecting item, especially during the crisis, but the proper and faultless use is also equally important. If hand sanitizer either homemade or commercial is misused, it cannot kill the maximum numbers of germs and the potential benefits will be lost. The type of a hand sanitizer is also very important because non-alcoholic hand sanitizers either homemade or commercial, cannot kill the bacteria and viruses too much extent. These debates will be covered in the next chapter.

# CHAPTER 2: DIFFERENT TYPES OF HAND SANITIZERS

The most important debate related to hand sanitizer is about its type and specifications. There are varieties of different hand sanitizers available commercially, and some types can also be made at home without a hassle. The type of hand sanitizer depends upon its alcoholic or non-alcoholic nature. It can be a liquid hand sanitizer or a foam hand sanitizer. It can also be divided as commercially made or homemade. Commercially made hand sanitizers and homemade hand sanitizers have no major differences. The differences lie only in the form of branding companies because all benefits can be achieved from a high quality homemade hand sanitizer. It is different to face masks. High quality homemade face mask is somewhat less superior to surgical mask produced commercially.

So, it is a smart bet to make one's own hand sanitizer at home rather than struggling to find a commercially made hand sanitizer from the markets especially during the periods of lockdown and crisis. Following are some major types of hand sanitizers:

**Classification on the basis of alcohol:**

*Alcoholic hand sanitizers:*

Alcoholic hand sanitizer, as the name implies is the type of hand sanitizer which has some type of alcohol in it. Alcohol is a potent antibacterial and antiviral agent which is used on a wide scale all over the world for disinfection purpose. The use of alcohol is not limited to hand sanitizer as it is used as community disinfectant in colonies, hospitals and large public areas as well. However, there are different types of alcohols. In hand sanitizer and high-quality homemade hand sanitizer, isopropanol alcohol or also called rubbing alcohol is used as the alcohol of choice. This alcohol is most potent in its bactericidal actions as well as it is less hazardous to the skin, which makes it a perfect choice to be used in hand sanitizer or high-quality homemade hand sanitizer. Methyl alcohol which is present in spirits, cannot be used in hand sanitizer or high-quality homemade hand sanitizer because it has methane which is not only toxic to the skin but it has a foul smell. Methane is added in methyl alcohol on purpose so that nobody can drink it.

A good commercial hand sanitizer or high-quality homemade hand sanitizer must have at least 90-95% concentrated isopropanol alcohol which combined with other ingredients becomes diluted. This diluted quantity should fall above 55-60% of the total concentration of a hand sanitizer or high-quality homemade hand sanitizer. This 60% or above the concentration of isopropanol alcohol is highly essential for the proper killing of bacteria and viruses from hands. Lower quantities will have fewer disinfectant benefits.

*Non-alcoholic hand sanitizers:*

These types of hand sanitizers contain no alcohol, and these are not actually the type of sanitizer. These types of products which contain bactericidal or disinfectant benzalkonium chloride and some antiviral agents are mostly used as home disinfectants rather than hand sanitizers. Much low-quality hand sanitizer, which is present in commercial markets, don't have alcohol in them. These types of hand sanitizers contain only glycerin and perfuming agents which are not ideal for disinfection purposes. They have very low to zero capacity of killing bacteria and viruses, and thus, these types of hand sanitizer should not be used. Hand sanitizers with non-alcoholic products can also cause harm to the skin because ethanol or isopropanol when used in a proper diluted amount, are skin-friendly and more bactericidal in nature.

**Classification on the basis of consistency:**

*Liquid hand sanitizers:*
These types of hand sanitizers are liquid in nature and easily absorbable in the skin. The most selling type of hand sanitizers is in liquid form. These types of hand sanitizers usually contain more than 80% of isopropanol or ethanol. Similarly, these types of hand sanitizers can be alcoholic or non-alcoholic as well as commercial or homemade. The consistency of liquid hand sanitizer is just like water. These are hand sanitizers of choice in the medical profession to disinfect the hands before operative procedures and surgeries.

*Gel hand sanitizers:*
These types of hand sanitizer contain aloe Vera or glycerin in it to make them more skin-friendly and numerous inconsistency. They are gel type in consistency as compared to liquid hand sanitizers.

These types of hand sanitizers contain 60-70% of isopropanol or rubbing alcohol and ideal for general use. High-quality homemade hand sanitizers are gel type inconsistency. Some perfuming agents can also be added in it to make it more cosmetic in nature. They are mostly clear without any colour.

*Foam hand sanitizers:*

These types of hand sanitizers are popular among medical professionals and mostly sold in large portable containers. These are not pocket type hand sanitizers. The consistency of these types of hand sanitizers is foamy and whitish in colour. They contain nearly 60-80% of isopropanol or ethanol and alcoholic in nature.

High-quality homemade hand sanitizers are not foamy type, and gel type hand sanitizer is mostly used as high-quality homemade hand sanitizer.

**Classification on the basis of production:**

Hand sanitizers can be commercially produced or homemade.

*Commercially produced hand sanitizers:*

The commercial type hand sanitizers are sold under different types of brand names. They are mass-produced types of hand sanitizer which are distributed worldwide. Many cosmetic and hygiene type industries also produced their commercial hand sanitizers. The price range of these types of hand sanitizers is varying and depends upon the brand and amount of the product. They can be large portable containers or pocket-sized bottles of commercially produced hand sanitizers. During the periods of pandemics and infectious crisis, these types of hand sanitizers suffer a lot because of increased consumption and decreased production, which leads to reduced or zero availability of these types of hand sanitizers. It can be an alarming situation because hand sanitization is the primary preventive strategy to control infectious transfer during the periods of crisis and emergencies related to global pandemics and epidemics. So, in those cases, high-quality homemade hand sanitizer can be a better substitute.

*High-quality homemade hand sanitizer:*

These types of hand sanitizers are not commercially made and can easily be manufactured at home by using minimal and items of daily use. These are alcoholic in nature and gel type inconsistency. It can be stored in a pocket-size bottle or in large containers. High-quality homemade hand sanitizer is the cheapest type of hand sanitizers and easiest to make. The quality of high-quality homemade hand sanitizers is never less than commercially-made hand sanitizers because high-quality homemade hand sanitizers contain all the necessary items which make them highly bactericidal and disinfectant in nature. The biggest benefit of high-quality homemade hand sanitizers is the availability during the periods of pandemics and crisis in which commercial production can be shaken to its core. During the periods of pandemics and infectious crisis, these types of hand sanitizers suffer a lot because of increased consumption and decreased production, which leads to reduced or zero availability of these types of hand sanitizers. It can be an alarming situation because hand sanitization is the primary preventive strategy to control infectious transfer during the periods of crisis and emergencies related to global pandemics and epidemics. So, in those cases, high-quality homemade hand sanitizer can be a better substitute.

The process of making a high-quality homemade hand sanitizer is straightforward and simple and requires items of daily household use. Only the alcohol should be purchased commercially, but isopropanol and ethanol are widely available on regular pharmacies even during the periods of pandemics. In the next chapters of this book, the details of production the high-quality homemade hand sanitizer will be discussed with relevant subheadings.

## CHAPTER 3: HOW TO MAKE HIGH-QUALITY HAND SANITIZER AT HOME WITH MINIMAL BURDEN:

The use of hand sanitizer during the period of crisis and the global pandemic is highly important because it is the best step in the prevention of deadly infections and transmission of diseases from one person to another. The use of commercial hand sanitizer for infectious control is no doubt essential and beneficial, but during the crisis and difficult lockdown situation, hand sanitizer which is commercially produced can be wiped off from the markets, but the need of using these hand sanitizers can increase every passing day of pandemic crisis. So, there should be some substitute for these commercially made hand sanitizers. The substitute should be equally beneficial and effective; it should be more readily available and easy to access; it must kill nearly 95-99% of bacteria and viruses, including pandemic infections.

Here lies a big question about the usefulness of high-quality homemade hand sanitizers. Does high-quality homemade hand sanitizer equally effective in killing the bacteria? The answer is a big yes because an alcohol-based high-quality homemade hand sanitizer can kill nearly 99% of bacteria and viruses similar to commercially made hand sanitizers. Another question is; does the high-quality homemade hand sanitizer can be readily available? The answer is again, yes because of the high-quality homemade hand sanitizer is very easy to make at home with the minimal burden and maximal benefits. It can be carried to anywhere in a pocket container, or it can be made in large quantities for the whole family. The third question in this regard is; does the high-quality homemade hand sanitizer cheap? YES! High-quality homemade hand sanitizer is much cheaper than the commercially made hand sanitizer.

These types of hand sanitizers are not commercially made and can easily be manufactured at home by using minimal and items of daily use. These are alcoholic in nature and gel type inconsistency. It can be stored in a pocket-size bottle or in large containers. High-quality homemade hand sanitizer is the cheapest type of hand sanitizers and easiest to make. The quality of high-quality homemade hand sanitizers is never less than commercially-made hand sanitizers because high-quality homemade hand sanitizers contain all the necessary items which make them highly bactericidal and disinfectant in nature. The biggest benefit of high-quality homemade hand sanitizers is the availability during the periods of pandemics and crisis in which commercial production can be shaken to its core. During the periods of pandemics and infectious crisis, these types of hand sanitizers suffer a lot because of increased consumption and decreased production, which leads to reduced or zero availability of these types of hand sanitizers. It can be an alarming situation because hand sanitization is the primary preventive strategy to control infectious transfer during the periods of crisis and emergencies related to global pandemics and epidemics. So, in those cases, high-quality homemade hand sanitizer can be a better substitute.

The process of making a high-quality homemade hand sanitizer is straightforward and simple and requires items of daily household use. Only the alcohol should be purchased commercially, but isopropanol and ethanol are widely available on regular pharmacies even during the periods of pandemics.

All it needs is the right quantity of 95% concentrated readily available isopropanol alcohol or ethanol, 20-30 ml of aloe Vera either natural or commercially produced, 25ml of pure glycerin and essential oil (12-14 drops) even few drops of lemon juice. These are all household items which are used for cosmetic purposes on a daily basis. There is no hectic preparation required to make a high-quality homemade hand sanitizer.

Next chapter will tell about the items required to make high-quality homemade hand sanitizer. For the convenience of readers, the process of high-quality homemade hand sanitizer production is divided into five straightforward steps.

**STEP 1: GATHERING THE REQUIRED ITEMS**

The first and initial step is to gather all the right supplies and items which can be utilized information of a high-quality homemade hand sanitizer. All it needs is the right quantity of 95% concentrated readily available isopropanol alcohol or ethanol, 20-30 ml of aloe Vera either natural or commercially produced, 25ml of pure glycerin and essential oil (12-14 drops) even few drops of lemon juice. These are all household items which are used for cosmetic purposes on a daily basis. There is no hectic preparation required to make a high-quality homemade hand sanitizer. Following are the items which will be used information of high-quality homemade hand sanitizer:

*The right type of alcohol:*

There are different types of alcohols which are used for multiple purposes. In high-quality homemade hand sanitizer, isopropanol alcohol or also called rubbing alcohol is used as the alcohol of choice. This alcohol is most potent in its bactericidal actions as well as it is less hazardous to the skin, which makes it a perfect choice to be used in hand sanitizer or high-quality homemade hand sanitizer. Methyl alcohol which is present in spirits, cannot be used in hand sanitizer or high-quality homemade hand sanitizer because it has methane which is not only toxic to the skin but it has a foul smell. Methane is added in methyl alcohol on purpose so that nobody can drink it.

A high-quality homemade hand sanitizer must have at least 90-95% concentrated isopropanol alcohol which, combined with other ingredients, becomes diluted. This diluted quantity should fall above 55-60% of the total concentration of a hand sanitizer or high-quality homemade hand sanitizer. This 60% or above a concentration of isopropanol alcohol is highly essential for the proper killing of bacteria and viruses from hands after mixing with other ingredients. Lower quantities will have fewer disinfectant benefits.

Isopropanol alcohol is also sold under the terminology of n-isopropanol, which is the isomer of basic type and has equal benefits. Ethanol is a precursor of ethyl-alcohol and sold under many brand names. The details about the chemistry of these types of alcohol will be baseless, and it will increase the complexity of the process. The take-home notes regarding alcohol use for the production of high-quality homemade hand sanitizer are:

- Use isopropanol or ethanol for high-quality homemade hand sanitizer
- Never use methyl alcohol or methylated spirit for this purpose
- The isolated alcohol concentration should be above 90% or ideally above 95%.
- Alcohol concentration after mixing with other ingredients should be above 60%

## Aloe Vera:

Aloe Vera is a plant which is available worldwide. The plant is very famous for its benefits in cosmetic purposes. This plant secretes a specific type of gel which is very sticky in nature and colourless. The actual cosmetic benefits of aloe Vera gel are because of this gel produced by the plant. It is very rich in vitamin especially vitamin E, vitamin A, vitamin K, vitamin B complex and to some extent vitamin C. This aloe Vera gel promotes softness in the skin and makes it smooth, shiny and wrinkle-free. Aloe Vera is very famous in its benefits to slow down the aging process of the skin. Aloe Vera gel is an essential component in high-quality homemade hand sanitizer because it acts as a stabilizing agent for alcohol. It helps in devolatilizing the isopropanol alcohol, which is called stabilization so that it can be used on the skin for the long term. Aloe Vera gel is itself a bactericidal agent to some extent.

The question regarding the use of aloe Vera gel is about its availability. Aloe Vera gel is readily available commercially as well as the natural sources of aloe Vera are rich in many countries of the world. This plant is easy to grow, and it requires no extra care. The best thing about this plant is it can be grown inside a living room as it requires less sunlight and it is an indoor type of plant. Moreover, s single leaf of aloe Vera plant can provide 10-15ml of gel quickly. Commercial availability of this gel is also straightforward, and crisis-related to pandemics and infectious diseases don't affect its commercial availability. It is readily available commercially in cheap rates. A standard container of commercially produced aloe

Vera gel contains nearly 300ml of gel but to make a high-quality homemade hand sanitizer; it requires the only 30ml of aloe Vera gel for 60ml of high-quality homemade hand sanitizer.

*Pure glycerin:*

Glycerin is a must-have item for every house. It has numerous benefits and uses. It is mostly used as a cosmetic product in routine cosmetic purposes. However, its medical uses are also extensive. The most significant benefit of pure glycerin is its healing capacity for skin and oral mucosa. This is the reason for the use of glycerin on blisters in the mouth and other areas of the body. Its specific chemistry makes it highly effective in healing the damages in skin. It is rich in vitamins and water, which makes it highly useful in proper hydration of the skin.

These benefits of pure glycerin make it an essential component in high-quality homemade hand sanitizer. High-quality homemade hand sanitizer contains alcohol which can harm the skin when used alone. However, adding aloe Vera gel and pure glycerin can reduce the skin-damaging side effects of alcohol too much extent. It is essential that the quantity of aloe Vera gel and glycerin should be well calculated. A 60ml high-quality homemade hand sanitizer should contain nearly 15ml of glycerin so that the overall quantity of isopropanol alcohol should stand well above 60% of the total mixture, which is highly essential for its bactericidal actions. The other benefit of pure glycerin is availability. It is commercially produced and readily available on pharmacies and cosmetic stores.

## *The essential oil of choice:*

Essential oils are extracted from various plants which have historical benefits and uses. There is a wide variety of essential oils, and nearly every type of essential oil is available in every part of any country. Some most essential types of essential oil are:

- Lavender
- Rosemary
- Olive oil
- Eucalyptus
- Rose
- Grapefruit
- Cedarwood

Any type of above mentioned or personally chosen essential oil can be used in high-quality homemade hand sanitizer. The purpose of essential oil in high-quality homemade hand sanitizer is to provide a soothing smell to the product so that it can be more useable. Use of essential oil is a personal choice. However, it is recommended to use any type of essential oil because:

1. It will provide a soothing smell to the product.
2. It will increase the usability of the product.
3. It will reduce the sharpness of the alcohol
4. Essential oils have their own bactericidal benefits
5. It is skin-friendly and heals the skin

In case, if an essential oil is unavailable, lemon juice or rose water can be used as a substitute. Almost 10-14 drops of essential oil will be needed to add soothing fragrance to high-quality homemade hand sanitizer.

*A measuring cup:*

A glass measuring cup is ideal to use for high-quality homemade hand sanitizer. It will help in calculating the exact amount of items which will be used in a high-quality homemade hand sanitizer. A proper concentration of every item is essential for the proper effectiveness of a high-quality homemade hand sanitizer.

*A bowl:*

A glass bowl is required to mix the calculated amounts of:
- Isopropanol alcohol
- Glycerin
- Aloe Vera gel
- Essential oil

*A spoon:*

A spoon or mixer is essential to mix all the items thoroughly in a bowl.

*A pocket-sized container with lid:*

Any type of pocket-sized plastic container with foldable lid is essential to store the high-quality homemade hand sanitizer. The container should have the capacity to be filled with 60-70ml of gel, high-quality homemade hand sanitizer.

Some specific qualities of an ideal container are as follows:
1. It should be a plastic container
2. It must have an easy to open/close yet the tight lid
3. It should have the capacity for 60-70ml of gel hand sanitizer
4. It should be clean and germ-free.
5. Any type of old hand sanitizer container can also be used.
6. It should be appropriately marked as a hand sanitizer to prevent any type of misuse.
7. It should be air-tight.
8. It should be leakage proof.

**Some additional items which can also be used:**

*Rosewater:*

It can be used as a substitute for glycerin or essential oil. The quantity should be no more than 20-30ml for a 70ml high-quality homemade hand sanitizer.

*Lemon juice:*

One tablespoon lemon juice can substitute 12-14 drops of essential oil

*Hydrogen peroxide:*

It should only be used when hand sanitizer is required in a large community.

## STEP 2: USING ALL THE NECESSARY PRECAUTIONS

High-quality homemade hand sanitizer is easy to make and safe to use. However, the process of making a high-quality homemade hand sanitizer contains some risks and necessary precautions are highly essential to avoid any type of mishap.

**Precautions related to use of alcohol:**

1. Alcohol is never a consumable item. Drinking alcohol can lead to a catastrophic crisis; even death can occur immediately.
2. Raw alcohol is highly damaging for skin, and its use can lead to blistering and rupture of skin. Even severe burns are also possible.
3. Methyl alcohol should never be used in high-quality homemade hand sanitizer because it contains methane which is highly toxic, foul-smelling and dangerous for skin.
4. Alcohol is a volatile agent, and keeping it in an open container is not a smart choice.
5. Alcohol is a highly inflammable material, and any type of inflammable gadget should be kept away from it.
6. Naked wires which can spark can also cause a fire if alcohol is present in close contact.
7. It is dangerous for eyes, and ideally, safety goggles and gloves should be used to avoid damages.

8. Alcohol should be kept away from open wounds and active infections as well as burned surfaces.
9. It should only be contained in a clean container.
10. It is colourless, and thus, it can be consumed by an unaware person.

**Precautions specific for children, old and disable population:**
1. Making high-quality homemade hand sanitizer is a risky job, and children, old and disable population should be kept away from it.
2. It is possible that children can consume hand sanitizer so it should be kept away from children.
3. Alcohol is colourless, and thus, it can be consumed by an unaware person.
4. Alcohol is a highly inflammable material, and any type of inflammable gadget should be kept away from it.

**Precautions related to use of container:**
1. It should be a plastic container
2. It must have an easy to open/close yet the tight lid
3. It should have the capacity for 60-70ml of gel hand sanitizer
4. It should be clean and germ-free.
5. Any type of old hand sanitizer container can also be used.
6. It should be appropriately marked as a hand sanitizer to prevent any type of misuse.
7. It should be air-tight.

8. It should be leakage proof.

**Precautions related to use of hydrogen peroxide:**
1. Hydrogen peroxide is a chemical, and it can cause blistering when applied to sensitive skin
2. Undiluted hydrogen peroxide is damaging for hands and skin.
3. Alcohol is a highly inflammable material, and any type of inflammable gadget should be kept away from it.
4. Hydrogen peroxide is never a consumable item. Drinking alcohol can lead to a catastrophic crisis; even death can occur immediately.
5. It is colourless, and thus, it can be consumed by an unaware person.

## STEP 3: MEASURING THE CALCULATED AMOUNT OF NECESSARY ITEMS:

The next step information of a high-quality homemade hand sanitizer is to measure the exact quantity of every item used. Measuring is essential because a high-quality homemade hand sanitizer must have at least 90-95% concentrated isopropanol alcohol which, combined with other ingredients, becomes diluted. This diluted quantity should fall above 55-60% of the total concentration of a hand sanitizer or high-quality homemade hand sanitizer. This 60% or above a concentration of isopropanol alcohol is highly essential for the proper killing of bacteria and viruses from hands after mixing with other ingredients. Lower quantities will have fewer disinfectant benefits. A glass measuring cup is ideal to use for high-quality homemade hand sanitizer. It will help in calculating the exact amount of items which will be used in a high-quality homemade hand sanitizer. A proper concentration of every item is essential for the proper effectiveness of a high-quality homemade hand sanitizer.

*Measuring alcohol:*

It can be started by using a glass measuring scale to measure 35-40ml of rubbing alcohol (isopropanol alcohol) or ethanol. The final product must have at least 60% alcohol concentration.

*Measuring the aloe Vera gel:*

Take the measuring glass and measure 25ml of aloe Vera gel. It will act as a stabilizing agent.

*Measuring the glycerin:*

Take pure glycerin and measure 10-15ml of its quantity by using a measuring scale

*Measuring the essential oil:*

Take 10-14 drops of essential oil in a separate cup.

## STEP 4: MIXING THE CALCULATED AMOUNT OF NECESSARY ITEMS

In the fourth step of high-quality homemade hand sanitizer, take the glass bowl which contains the measured quantities of:

- Isopropanol alcohol 35-40ml
- Glycerin 10ml
- Aloe Vera gel 25ml
- Essential oil 14 drops

Use the spoon or a butter mixture to mix the solution thoroughly and adequately. The final product should be a vicious type of non-sticky gel.

The final product will contain 60% or more concentration of isopropanol alcohol. High-quality homemade hand sanitizer must have at least 90-95% concentrated isopropanol alcohol which, combined with other ingredients, becomes diluted. This diluted quantity should fall above 55-60% of the total concentration of a hand sanitizer or high-quality homemade hand sanitizer. This 60% or above a concentration of isopropanol alcohol is highly essential for the proper killing of bacteria and viruses from hands after mixing with other ingredients.

Now the high-quality homemade hand sanitizer is prepared. This recipe of making hand sanitizer at home has strengths of being accessible and affordable. It requires no cumbersome arrangement or unique items which can be hard to find during the periods of crisis and pandemics. It is the cheapest type of hand sanitizer, yet it contains the maximum capacity to kill almost 99% of bacteria and viruses. It can be the best substitute of commercially made hand sanitizers which can be unavailable during the periods of lockdown and pandemics.

## STEP 5: HOW TO STORE IN SAFE AND USEABLE CONTAINER

Any type of pocket-sized plastic container with foldable lid is essential to store the high-quality homemade hand sanitizer. The container should have the capacity to be filled with 60-70ml of gel, high-quality homemade hand sanitizer.

Some specific qualities of an ideal container are as follows:

1. It should be a plastic container
2. It must have an easy to open/close yet the tight lid
3. It should have the capacity for 60-70ml of gel hand sanitizer
4. It should be clean and germ-free.
5. Any type of old hand sanitizer container can also be used.
6. It should be appropriately marked as a hand sanitizer to prevent any type of misuse.
7. It should be air-tight.
8. It should be leakage proof.

A high-quality container is essential to store a high-quality homemade hand sanitizer because it will prevent it from contamination and volatilization. A broken, leaked, or contaminated container can minimize the effects of high-quality homemade hand sanitizer so it should be selected smartly.

This is the last step of making a high-quality hand sanitizer at home. In the next chapter, some other less famous yet easy recipes of homemade hand sanitizer will be discussed.

# CHAPTER 4: SPECIFIC RECIPE OF MAKING HAND SANITIZER FOR LARGER POPULATION:

There is an international guideline related to making a hand sanitizer for a large population which can serve in crisis and helps in the prevention of deadly diseases when there is no other available resource left.

It is much similar to the above-mentioned technique. However, the effectiveness of this type of hand sanitizer can be somewhat lower to above mentioned high-quality homemade hand sanitizer because it is made in bulk and proper 2:1 ratio of isopropanol alcohol to other ingredients is tough to maintain in this bulk production.

Items with specific quantities for this bulk produced hand sanitizer are:

*Isopropanol alcohol:*

As mentioned above, the best choice to make any type of alcohol hand sanitizer is to use isopropanol or rubbing alcohol. Ethanol can also be used. The final product will contain 60% or more concentration of isopropanol alcohol. High-quality homemade hand sanitizer must have at least 90-95% concentrated isopropanol alcohol which combined with other ingredients becomes diluted, and it is same for bulk produced hand sanitizer. This diluted quantity should fall above 55-60% of the total concentration of a hand sanitizer or high-quality homemade hand sanitizer. This 60% or above a concentration of isopropanol alcohol is highly essential for the proper killing of bacteria and viruses from hands after mixing with other ingredients.

### *Hydrogen peroxide:*

Hydrogen peroxide is used as 1:2 with the alcohol, which means nearly half quantity of hydrogen peroxide is used as compared to alcohol. The uniqueness of this type of mass-produced hand sanitizer is the use of hydrogen peroxide along with the alcohol to save time and resources.

### *Glycerol:*

Pure glycerol is used in 0.5/2 ratio, that means the only quarter concentration of glycerol will be used as compared to alcohol to prevent the dilution below 60%.

### *Distil water or boiled cold water:*

Distil water or boiled cold water is used in 0.5/2 ratio that means only a quarter concentration of water will be used as compared to alcohol to prevent the dilution below 60%.

# CHAPTER 5: SPECIAL CONSIDERATIONS ON USING HOMEMADE HAND SANITIZER:

During the intense periods of lockdowns and global epidemics, the use of hand sanitizer increases to nearly 700% of ordinary days. The production declines to nearly 60-70% for this essential preventive item. So this disturbed consumption to production ratio causes much distress among the human population, which at that time may be fighting with a disease without any possible cure and high spread rate. In that case, only prevention can help in controlling the numbers of affected individuals.

So, in this stressful situation, high-quality homemade hand sanitizer can be the best substitute which is cheapest and yet the most effective in killing 99% of bacteria and viruses. It takes no special requirements or very hefty amount to produce a high-quality homemade hand sanitizer. Homemade face mask and high-quality homemade hand sanitizer, when used together, can prevent nearly 100% transmission of deadly infections to or from any person, and unlike the homemade face mask, high-quality homemade hand sanitizer is equally beneficial as the commercially produced hand sanitizer.

Apart from these tremendous benefits, there are some special considerations related to high-quality homemade hand sanitizer which should be noted about a high-quality homemade hand sanitizer to prevent any mishap and to increase the effectiveness of high-quality homemade hand sanitizer to its maximum. These considerations related to high-quality homemade hand sanitizer include proper use of high-quality homemade hand sanitizer and proper care of high-quality homemade hand sanitizer.

*Proper use of high-quality homemade hand sanitizer:*

- High-quality homemade hand sanitizer can only be effective when applied correctly.
- Take 2-3 drops on your fist.
- Rub both hands in circular motions.
- Rub between the fingers
- Rub the nail beds of one hand of the palm of other hand and vice versa.
- Apply thoroughly on the back of hands too.
- Also, apply over the wrist portion.
- Consume at least 30 seconds in applying the high-quality homemade hand sanitizer on hands
- It takes 60 seconds for a high-quality homemade hand sanitizer to kill nearly 99% of bacteria and viruses
- Don't eat immediately after the application of high-quality homemade hand sanitizer because alcohol can cause disturbances in the mouth.
- Avoid rubbing eyes after application of high-quality homemade hand sanitizer for at least 10 minutes.
- Rinse your eyes or mouth thoroughly with water if feeling itching and discomfort.
- When available, I always prefer hand washing or hand sanitization.

- Keep safe from the reach of children.
- Keep in a safe and clean place
- Alcohol is inflammable, and thus it should never be used near fire
- Avoid doing tasks which require flame-like cooking, smoking etc. after application of high-quality homemade hand sanitizer because it can catch fire for at least 5 minutes after application.
- For testing purpose, pour a drop of high-quality homemade hand sanitizer on the floor and apply flame to it. Hand sanitizer will catch the flame, and if a paper is brought near it, it will adequately burn. So safety is essential.
- Never use methyl alcohol or methylated spirit for high-quality homemade hand sanitizer because it is not ideal for it.
- Always use clean and leakage proof container to keep the hand sanitizer safe.
- Don't waste the precious items as well as high-quality homemade hand sanitizer because, during a crisis, nearly 40% of the human population doesn't have access to this essential item.
- Contact with a doctor immediately if any unresolvable problem occurs.

# CHAPTER 6: PROPER HANDWASHING TECHNIQUE:

The global health authorities have provided clear guidelines on proper techniques of handwashing. Handwashing with soap is superior to hand sanitization and when possible, always prefer washing hands thoroughly with soap over hand sanitization with high-quality homemade hand sanitizer.

There are six steps of proper handwashing technique and hand should be washed for at least 20 seconds with disinfectant soap so that maximum number of deadly bacteria and viruses can be killed.

Take soup on wet hand and:
1. Rub the palms with each other
2. Rub between fingers from the palmar side
3. Rub between fingers from the back of the hands
4. Rub the nail beds on palms
5. Rub between the thumbs
6. Rub on the back of hands, including the wrists.

By using these six steps for handwashing and hand sanitization, maximum numbers of bacteria and viruses can be killed effectively.

## Summary:

Hand sanitization means clearing hands from germs which can be bacteria, viruses, spores or fungi, which can cause infections by penetrating through the human body and start chains of reactions which lead to full-fledged diseases. Hand washing and hand sanitization are always misinterpreted as the same in respect of terminology and meaning. However, technically speaking, hand washing and hand sanitization are very different from one another. The unavailability of hand sanitizers during infectious pandemics can be more dangerous to pandemic itself. The most important strategy used by health authorities during pandemics and epidemics is to prevent the incurable and poorly controlled infections rather than treating them.

Homemade hand sanitizers are natural to make and more readily available than the commercially made hand sanitizers. The effectiveness and mode of action of homemade hand sanitizers are hundred per cent the same as compared to commercially made hand sanitizers. It is important to check the quality, techniques and item used in homemade hand sanitizer to achieve the maximum antibacterial and antiviral activity. Homemade hand sanitizer when entirely made and used can kill nearly 99% of bacteria and viruses in a single go when it is used for more than 20 seconds on hands. Hand sanitizers are classified on the basis of types, formation, production and usage.

Making high-quality homemade hand sanitizer is secure, and all it needs is the right quantity of 95% concentrated readily available isopropanol alcohol or ethanol, 20-30 ml of aloe Vera either natural or commercially produced, 25ml of pure glycerin and few drops of essential oil of your choice or even few drops of lemon juice. These are all household items which are used for cosmetic purposes on a daily basis. There is no hectic preparation required to make a high-quality homemade hand sanitizer.

There are five steps in making of high-quality homemade hand sanitizers.

- Step 1: gathering the required items
- Step 2: using all the necessary precautions
- Step 3: measuring the calculated amount of necessary items
- Step 4: mixing the calculated amount of necessary items
- Step 5: how to store in a safe and useable container

Apart from these great benefits, there are some special considerations related to high-quality homemade hand sanitizer which are essentially about a high-quality homemade hand sanitizer to prevent any mishap and to increase the effectiveness of high-quality homemade hand sanitizer to its maximum. The global health authorities have provided clear guidelines on proper techniques of handwashing. Handwashing with soap is superior to hand sanitization and when possible, always prefer washing hands thoroughly with soap over hand sanitization with high-quality homemade hand sanitizer. There are six steps of proper handwashing technique and hand should be washed for at least 20 seconds with disinfectant soap so that maximum number of deadly bacteria and viruses can be killed.

1. Rub the palms with each other
2. Rub between fingers from the palmar side
3. Rub between fingers from the back of the hands
4. Rub the nail beds on palms
5. Rub between the thumbs
6. Rub on the back of hands, including the wrists.

www.ingramcontent.com/pod-product-compliance
Lightning Source LLC
Chambersburg PA
CBHW050319220526
45465CB00005B/2053